MORNING WORKOUT FOR OLDER MEN

*7 Simple Stretching Exercise
for Seniors
To gain Balance, Stability and
improve Body Postures*

Corey M. Clark

TABLE OF CONTENT

INTRODUCTION

In the center of a bustling city, among the ebb and flow of metropolitan life, lived Jerome, a man whose journey from the depths of health issues to the pinnacle of vigor exemplifies the power of resolve and endurance.

Jerome's story of change occurred against a backdrop of difficulty as he dealt with a slew of health challenges that threatened to eclipse his zest for living.

Jerome struggled to walk, as if weighed down by unseen weights tying him to the ground, navigating a landscape filled with joint problems that challenged his stamina and dampened his soul.

His once-simple mobility now resembled a delicate dance on a tightrope, with each wobbly stride putting his balance at risk.

Despite the huge challenges that lay ahead of him, Jerome refused to give up. With unyielding commitment as his guiding light, he set out on a search for answers that promised to enlighten the route to regeneration.

During his search for answers, Jerome came across a guide—a light of hope in the shadows—who provided a road map to fresh vigor.

Armed with this unexpected resource, Jerome started on a transformative journey that defied the odds and changed the course of his life.

The guide became his compass, guiding him through a maze of wellness measures carefully suited to his specific health challenges.

From food changes that fed his body from inside to targeted activities that strengthened his muscles and restored his balance, Jerome welcomed each suggestion with a resolute commitment to recapture his energy.

As the days progressed into weeks and weeks into months, Jerome witnessed a miraculous transformation inside himself.

The shackles that had formerly bound him were released, allowing him to move freely once again. Joint pains subsided as a result of attentive self-care, and his formerly unstable equilibrium regained stability on a firm foundation of resilience.

With each passing day, Jerome's steps became more confident, his movements more fluid, and his mood more buoyant. Liberated from the confines of his health problems, he embraced life with boundless enthusiasm. From leisurely strolls through sun-kissed parks to adventurous exploits that took him beyond his comfort zone, Jerome relished the simple delight of living life to the fullest.

Today, when he looks at the chapters of his life, Jerome is a living witness to the power of perseverance, persistence, and unflinching faith in the potential of change.

His narrative serves as a light of hope for everyone who is navigating the maze of health issues, reminding them that amid the depths of hardship lies the germ of resilience, ready to bloom and illuminate the route to a life lived in vibrant harmony with vigor and joy.

Chapter 1: The Science Behind Morning Exercise

Morning exercise has long been advocated as a positive habit for both physical and mental health. Understanding the science underlying this technique explains why it's so powerful.

1. Hormonal Response: Exercising in the morning causes the release of endorphins, neurotransmitters that improve mood and reduce stress levels.

Furthermore, morning exercise can help control cortisol levels, the stress hormone, resulting in improved stress management throughout the day.

2. Metabolic Boost: Physical exercise in the morning boosts metabolism, which aids in weight management and fat loss. This mechanism, known as excess post-exercise oxygen consumption (EPOC), permits the body to continue burning calories at a high rate long after the activity has ended.

3. *Improved Focus and Cognitive Function:* Morning exercise boosts cognitive function and mental clarity by boosting blood flow to the brain. This increase in circulation provides oxygen and nutrients, increasing alertness and attention for work throughout the day.

4. *Consistency and regimen:* Creating a morning workout regimen encourages discipline and consistency. Individuals who start the day with physical activity are more likely to stick to their fitness objectives and live an active lifestyle.

5. *Improved Sleep Quality:* Unlike the popular belief that exercising in the evening affects sleep, morning exercise has been demonstrated to increase sleep quality. It modulates the circadian clock, encouraging deeper and more restorative sleep cycles at night.

6.   *Improved   Mood   and   Well-Being:* Morning exercise promotes general well-being by lowering symptoms of anxiety and despair. Physical activity and exposure to natural light early in the day improve mood and energy levels.

7. Appetite Regulation: Morning exercise can help moderate your appetite throughout the day. According to research, those who exercise in the morning eat better and have fewer desires for bad foods.

8. Increased Productivity: Starting the day with exercise establishes a pleasant tone and increases productivity. Physical activity increases the release of neurotransmitters such as dopamine and serotonin, which are linked to motivation and goal-directed behavior.

The research behind early exercise demonstrates its multiple advantages for physical, mental, and emotional health. Individuals who include regular morning workouts in their routines might improve their overall health and productivity throughout the day.

Mental and Physical Health Benefits

Mental and physical health are inextricably linked, especially among seniors. Participating in activities that boost both areas of health can considerably increase the overall well-being of older people. Regular physical exercise is essential for elders' physical well-being.

It improves strength, flexibility, balance, and endurance, lowering the chance of falls and injuries. physical activity produces endorphins, which are neurotransmitters that boost happiness while decreasing tension and anxiety.

Remaining physically active might have a favorable impact on mental health. Seniors who exercise on a daily basis frequently have better cognitive function and are less likely to develop dementia. Exercise increases the synthesis of brain-derived neurotrophic factor (BDNF), which aids in the growth and maintenance of brain cells. This can result in improved memory, attention, and general cognitive performance in seniors.

In addition to physical activity, maintaining social relationships and participating in cerebral stimulation are essential for seniors' mental health.

Social connection can help reduce feelings of loneliness and isolation, which are frequent in older persons and can lead to melancholy and anxiety. Joining groups, volunteering, or taking part in group activities can give possibilities for social interaction and support.

Mental stimulation, such as solving puzzles, reading, or learning new skills, is essential for keeping the mind fresh and cognitively functioning. Seniors who engage in cognitively challenging activities are more likely to retain cognitive talents and lower their risk of cognitive decline as they age.

Prioritizing both physical and mental health is critical for elders to maintain a good standard of living. Regular physical exercise, social interaction, and mental stimulation can all help older persons maintain their physical and mental health.

By adding these activities into their daily routines, seniors can improve their physical health, cognitive function, and overall pleasure and contentment. Taking care of both the body and the mind is essential for aging gracefully and having a high quality of life in later years.

Overcoming Common Obstacles

Starting an early fitness regimen can be difficult, especially for older men who may encounter specific challenges.

However, with the correct solutions, these challenges may be overcome, resulting in a healthier and more active lifestyle. Here are some typical hurdles and how to deal with them:

1. Lack of Motivation: Getting up early to exercise can be challenging, especially if motivation is low. To combat this, establish defined and attainable goals. Whether it's increasing strength, flexibility, or general health, having a clear goal may offer the drive to get out of bed.

2. Joint Pain and Stiffness: Aging frequently causes joint pain and stiffness, making exercise difficult. Prioritize low-impact activities like swimming, cycling, and yoga. These exercises help increase mobility and flexibility without placing undue strain on the joints.

3. *Fatigue:* Older men may feel more tired, making it difficult to stick to early workouts. Maintain a consistent sleep schedule and establish a pleasant nighttime ritual to promote good sleep hygiene. Consume healthy foods and remain hydrated to combat weariness.

4. *Time constraints:* Juggling job, family, and other responsibilities often leave little time for exercise. Incorporate brief and effective workouts that may be completed at home or at a local park. High-intensity interval training (HIIT) and circuit training are excellent ways to save time while also receiving a full-body workout.

5. *Lack of Equipment:* Older men who do not have access to a gym or pricey equipment may avoid exercising. Focus on bodyweight exercises that require little or no equipment, such as push-ups, squats, lunges, and planks. These workouts may be tailored to different fitness levels and are helpful for increasing strength and endurance.

6. *Weather Conditions:* Extreme weather might make it difficult to exercise outside. Prepare a backup plan for indoor exercises, such as watching internet workout videos or purchasing home gym equipment like resistance bands or dumbbells. Alternatively, join a local gym or community center for indoor exercise.

7. *Injury Risk:* Because older men are more likely to sustain injuries, it is critical to emphasize safety. Begin with a full warm-up to prepare the body for activity, and use correct stretching methods to avoid injuries. Listen to your body and don't push yourself too hard, especially while attempting new workouts.

By overcoming these frequent challenges with persistence and a proactive mentality, older men may effectively develop and maintain a morning fitness regimen that benefits their general health and well-being. Remember, consistency is essential, so stay focused and enjoy minor triumphs along the way.

Chapter 2: Setting the Stage: Preparing for Your Morning Routine

Establishing a daily routine sets the tone for the day, increasing productivity and general well-being, particularly among older men. Here's a quick approach to getting ready for your daily routine, with a focus on including an early workout:

1. Plan Ahead: Before you go to bed, put out your training clothing and any necessary equipment. Having everything ready saves time and prevents excuses in the morning.

2. Get Up Early: Aim to wake up at least 30 minutes to an hour before your workout time. This allows for a gradual awakening without haste.

3. Hydration: Start your day with a glass of water to help your body rehydrate after a long night of sleep. Proper hydration is vital for peak performance in your early workout.

4. Perform an active warm-up to get your muscles and joints ready for exercise. This can involve arm circles, leg swings, and modest stretches for main muscle groups.

5. Cardiovascular activity: Perform 15-20 minutes of cardiovascular activity to raise your heart rate and improve blood circulation. Brisk walking, cycling, and jumping jacks are also possible options.

6. Strength Training: Use resistance workouts that target various muscle areas. To increase efficiency, use compound motions like squats, lunges, push-ups, and rows.

7. Flexibility: Set aside time for stretching activities to increase flexibility and avoid injury. Hold each stretch for 15-30 seconds, with an emphasis on tight regions such the hamstrings, shoulders, and lower back.

8. Cool Down: After your workout, take a little cool-down session to gradually reduce your heart rate and relax your muscles. Gentle walking or cycling at a slower speed might aid healing.

9. Post-Workout Nutrition: To assist muscle regeneration and refill energy stores, refuel your body with a well-balanced post-workout meal or snack rich in protein and carbs.

10. Relax and Recovery: Give your body enough time to relax and recuperate in between workouts. Aim for 48 hours of recuperation time for each muscle group before addressing them again.

By implementing these steps into your morning routine, you can efficiently prepare for a productive exercise that will set a great tone for the rest of your day. Remember to listen to your body and modify your program as necessary to meet any physical restrictions or health issues.

With consistency and devotion, you may gain the many advantages of a morning workout designed specifically for older guys.

Establishing a Consistent Wake-Up Routine

A regular morning routine sets the tone for the whole day, affecting productivity, attitude, and general well-being. Here's how to create and keep a schedule that works for you:

Set a Specific Wake-Up Time: Select a time that provides you enough rest, usually between 6 and 8 hours of sleep every night. Consistency is essential here; attempt to get up at the same time every day, including weekends.

Establish a nighttime routine: A regular nighttime routine indicates to your body that it's time to relax. This might involve reading, meditating, or practicing relaxation techniques.

Limit Screen Time Before Bed: Screens produce blue light, which can interrupt your sleep cycle. To improve sleep quality, avoid using screens for at least an hour before bedtime.

Optimize Your Sleep Environment: Make sure your bedroom is dark, quiet, and at a suitable temperature. Invest on a comfy mattress and pillows to promote healthy sleep.

Avoid Stimulants Before Bedtime: Caffeine and nicotine might disrupt your ability to fall asleep. Limit your usage of these drugs in the hours before bedtime.

Use an Alarm Clock Wisely: While alarms are useful for getting up on time, use a moderate, non-invasive alarm tone to prevent being startled awake. Place your alarm clock across the room to avoid snooze button misuse.

Get Moving: Add some modest physical activity to your morning routine to wake up your body and mind. This might be as easy as stretching, yoga, or taking a brief stroll.

Expose Yourself to Natural Light: Natural light regulates your body's natural clock, suggesting when it's time to get up. As soon as you wake up, open your curtains or go a few minutes outside.

Stay Consistent: Consistency is essential for getting the advantages of a wake-up ritual. Stick to your pattern even on days when you would want to sleep in.

Listen to your body: Pay attention to how your body reacts to your wake-up routine and make changes as necessary. Everyone's sleep requirements are unique, so discover what works best for you.

Establishing and keeping to a consistent wake-up ritual will help you feel more energized, productive, and fulfilled throughout the day.

Nutrition Strategies for Morning Workouts

Beginning your day with a morning workout will boost your metabolism, promote alertness, and establish a positive tone for the day. Proper nutrition prior to and after these activities is critical for peak performance and recovery. Here are some thorough and simple nutritional strategies to consider:

1. Pre-workout nutrition:

Hydration: Start your day by drinking water to help your body rehydrate after a night's sleep. Drink at least 8-16 ounces of water 30 minutes before your workout to stay hydrated.

carbs: Eat readily digested carbs such as fruits, whole grains, or a modest amount of oatmeal to provide your body instant energy. Avoid meals that are heavy or rich in fiber, as they may cause discomfort when exercising.

Protein: A modest quantity of protein can assist repair and grow muscle tissue. Yogurt, almonds, and a protein smoothie are all convenient options.

Timing: To properly fuel your body for your workout, consume a small breakfast or snack containing carbs and protein around 1-2 hours before.

2. During exercise:

Hydration: Drink water during your workout to stay hydrated. If your workout is strenuous or lasts more than 60 minutes, use an electrolyte-containing sports drink to restore lost fluids.

3. Post-workout nutrition:

carbs: Within 30 minutes to an hour after finishing your workout, refuel your glycogen reserves with a combination of carbs and protein.

A banana with peanut butter, a turkey sandwich on whole-grain bread, or a protein smoothie with fruit will all help you refill your energy resources.

Protein: Include protein in your post-workout meal or snack to help with muscle repair and development. Greek yogurt, eggs, poultry, and tofu are all wonderful options.

Timing: To maximize recovery, eat a balanced breakfast or snack that includes carbs and protein within the post-workout interval.

4. *General Considerations:*

Listen to your body. Pay attention to how different meals make you feel before, during, and after you exercise. Experiment with different times and meal options to see what works best for your body.

Consistency: Sticking to a pre- and post-workout eating program will help you improve your performance and recuperation over time.

By using these complete dietary recommendations, you may successfully feed your body for morning workouts, maximize performance, and promote recovery for continuous progress toward your fitness objectives.

For individualized dietary recommendations, visit a healthcare practitioner or a certified dietitian.

Importance of Hydration and Pre-Workout Supplements

Hydration is critical for seniors, particularly while participating in vigorous activities such as exercise. As we age, our bodies become less effective in retaining water, making dehydration a major worry.

Staying hydrated is vital for general health and well-being since it helps with digestion, circulation, temperature control, and joint lubrication.

Seniors are more likely to become dehydrated during exercise due to diminished thirst sense and a deterioration in renal function. Proper hydration helps elders retain cognitive function, avoid muscular cramps, and lowers their risk of heat-related disorders.

Seniors should consume water before, during, and after exercise to restore lost fluids and electrolytes.

Pre-workout vitamins can also help seniors gain energy and improve performance. However, it is critical to pick supplements carefully and check with a healthcare practitioner before beginning any new regimen.

Seniors should search for supplements like caffeine, beta-alanine, and creatine, which have been proved to boost endurance, strength, and mental concentration.

Seniors should also be wary of supplements that include excessive levels of stimulants or needless ingredients, since they might aggravate pre-existing health concerns or conflict with prescriptions.

Natural alternatives, such as beetroot juice or sour cherry juice, can offer similar advantages without the hazards associated with certain pills.

Incorporating water and pre-workout vitamins into a senior's exercise regimen can greatly improve their general health and quality of life. Seniors may keep their independence, lower their risk of injury, and live a more active lifestyle if they stay hydrated and adequately nourished.

Seniors should listen to their bodies and tailor their water and supplement consumption to their specific needs and activity levels. It is critical to monitor any changes in thirst, urine color, or energy levels, since these might be signs of dehydration or insufficient fuelling.

Hydration and pre-workout vitamins are critical in helping seniors maintain their health and fitness. Seniors who prioritize appropriate hydration and incorporate safe and effective supplements into their regimen can improve their performance, lower their risk of injury, and get the advantages of regular exercise long into their golden years.

Chapter 3: Dynamic Warm-up Exercises for Older Men

Older men should perform dynamic warm-up activities to prepare their bodies for physical activity and lower the chance of injury. As men age, their muscles, joints, and ligaments become less flexible and more susceptible to injury.

An active warm-up program promotes blood flow, muscular flexibility, and joint mobility. Here's a complete and straightforward introduction to energetic warm-up activities for older guys.

Neck Rotations: Gently rotate your neck clockwise and counterclockwise to release the neck muscles and increase range of motion.

Arm Circles: Stand tall with your arms out to the sides. Rotate your arms in tiny circles, gradually increasing their size. This exercise relaxes the shoulder joints and increases blood circulation.

Shoulder Rolls: Roll your shoulders backward in a circular manner for 10–15 repetitions before reversing direction. This exercise lowers shoulder strain and increases flexibility.

Hip Circles: Stand with feet hip-width apart and hands on hips. Rotate your hips in a circular manner, progressively increasing the size of each circle. This workout increases hip mobility and flexibility.

Leg Swings: Use a firm surface for support. Swing one leg forth and backward in a controlled manner, then switch to the opposite leg. This exercise increases flexibility in the hamstrings and hip flexors.

Knee Raises: Stand tall and raise one knee to your chest, then repeat with the other knee. This exercise increases hip mobility and warms up the lower body muscles.

Ankle Circles: Sit on the edge of a chair, feet off the ground. Your ankles should be rotated in counterclockwise and clockwise direction

This exercise increases ankle mobility while decreasing the incidence of ankle injury.

Walking Lunges: Take a stride forward with one leg and bend both knees to lower yourself into a lunge stance. Push back to the starting position, then repeat with the other leg. This workout increases lower-body strength and flexibility.

High Knees: Stand tall and bring one knee to your chest while hopping on the other foot. Alternate knees when marching. This exercise elevates the heart rate and prepares the body for more strenuous exertion.

Trunk Rotations: Stand shoulder-width apart, hands on hips. Rotate your torso side to side while keeping your hips steady. This exercise increases spinal mobility and warms the core muscles.

Incorporating these dynamic warm-up exercises into your workout program can help older men prepare their bodies for physical activity, lower their chance of injury, and enhance their general flexibility and mobility. To avoid overexertion, start cautiously and raise the intensity gradually.

Joint Mobility and Flexibility Exercises

Joint mobility and flexibility exercises are vital components of any comprehensive fitness regimen. They improve general joint health, lower the chance of injury, and boost sports performance.

These exercises are designed to improve joint range of motion while also developing muscle, tendon, and ligament flexibility.

Incorporating these exercises into your normal training routine can result in better posture, more effective mobility, and a general sense of well-being.

Advantages of Joint Mobility and Flexibility Exercises:

Improved Range of Motion: Regularly completing joint mobility exercises will help you maintain and even expand your joint range of motion. This is essential for everyday tasks, including bending, reaching, and twisting.

Injury Prevention: Flexible muscles and joints are less vulnerable to injury. Flexibility exercises can help you avoid strains, sprains, and other common problems.

Enhanced Performance: Increased flexibility improves movement efficiency and performance in a variety of physical activities, including sports and exercise regimens. Coordination and balance can be enhanced

Better Posture: Tight muscles can cause bad posture. Flexibility exercises serve to lengthen muscles and improve posture, lowering the risk of discomfort and suffering caused by wrong alignment.

Reduced muscular Tension: Stretching and mobility exercises can help relieve muscular tension and increase relaxation, resulting in better stress management and general relaxation.

Below are kinds of flexibility and Joint Exercises respectively

Dynamic stretching is going through a range of motion to gently stretch muscles and improve flexibility. Examples include arm circles, leg swings, and trunk twists.

Static stretching is the practice of keeping a stretch posture for a certain amount of time, usually 15-30 seconds. This improves flexibility and may be done on a variety of muscle groups, including hamstrings, quadriceps, and shoulders.

Foam rolling, also known as self-myofascial release, involves applying pressure on tight muscles to relieve stress. It can assist to increase flexibility and minimize muscular pain.

Mobility exercises aim to improve joint function and range of motion through controlled motions. Examples include shoulder circles, hip circles, and ankle rotations.

Incorporating joint mobility and flexibility exercises into your workout program can help you move more effectively, minimize injury risk, and improve overall physical performance.

Whether you're an athlete wanting to enhance your game or just want to improve your joint health, these exercises are a great complement to any training routine.

Low-Impact Cardiovascular Warm-ups

Low-impact cardiovascular warm-ups are vital for getting your body ready for exercise while reducing stress on your joints and muscles.

These easy yet effective workouts raise heart rate, boost blood circulation, and relax muscles, laying the groundwork for a good training session.

Whether you're recuperating from an injury, have joint concerns, or simply prefer a gentler approach, including low-impact warm-ups in your workout regimen can offer a number of advantages.

Advantages of Low-Impact Cardiovascular Warm-ups:

Reduced Joint Stress: Low-impact warm-ups include motions that are soft on the joints, making them appropriate for people who have joint discomfort or arthritis. These exercises lubricate the joints and increase flexibility while avoiding unnecessary strain.

Improved Circulation: Low-impact cardiovascular warm-ups boost blood flow to the muscles, providing oxygen and nutrients required for peak performance. Enhanced circulation also supports speedier muscle recovery after an exercise.

Low-impact warm-ups progressively increase heart rate and body temperature, preparing muscles, tendons, and ligaments for more intensive exercise and lowering the risk of strains, sprains, and other injuries.

Enhanced Mobility: Including low-impact motions like walking, cycling, or swimming in your warm-up regimen enhances joint mobility and range of motion, making it simpler to complete exercises correctly.

Examples of Low-impact Cardiovascular Warm-ups:

Brisk Walking: A simple but efficient warm-up, brisk walking progressively raises heart rate while exercising several muscle groups. Begin at a relaxed pace and progressively increase speed to raise the intensity.

Stationary Cycling: Cycling on a stationary bike is a low-impact warm-up that works the lower body muscles while increasing cardiovascular fitness. Adjust the resistance and speed to your fitness level.

Swimming is a great low-impact warm-up that works the entire body while putting less strain on the joints. Swimming laps or other modest water activities will help raise heart rate and warm up muscles.

Elliptical training is a low-impact alternative to running or jogging that provides a full-body workout while reducing pressure on the knees and hips.

Incorporating these low-impact cardiovascular warm-ups into your exercise program will help you get the most out of your workout while reducing the chance of injury.

Whether you're prepared for strength training, endurance activities, or just want to keep active, a thorough warm-up is essential for a safe and productive workout.

Muscle Activation Drills for Injury Prevention

As we age, maintaining functional strength and mobility becomes increasingly important for a great quality of life. Muscle activation drills are critical tools for seniors to avoid injuries, improve stability, and keep independence in their everyday tasks.

These workouts focus on particular muscle areas to promote activation, ensure optimal movement patterns, and lower the risk of injuries and falls.

1. Significance of Muscle Activation Drills:

Muscle weakness and poor neuromuscular control are common in seniors, resulting in unbalanced movement patterns and an increased vulnerability to injury.

muscular activation workouts help elders restore and maintain muscular function by activating specific muscles, increasing joint stability, and improving general mobility.

2. Major Muscle Groups to Target:

Core Muscles: Exercises that target the core muscles (abdominals, obliques, and lower back) improve posture, balance, and spinal stability, lowering the risk of falling and injury.

Lower Body Muscles: Strengthening workouts for the quadriceps, hamstrings, glutes, and calves improve mobility, stability, and gait mechanics, which are essential for tasks such as walking and climbing stairs.

Upper Body Muscles: Working on muscles in the shoulders, back, and arms increases upper body strength, posture, and functional actions such as reaching and lifting.

3. Example Muscle Activation Drills:

Planks: Holding a plank posture works the core muscles, which promotes stability and spinal alignment.

Squats: Bodyweight squats or squats with tension bands work the lower body muscles, increasing balance and mobility.

Shoulder Retraction: Pulling the shoulder blades together engages the upper back muscles, which corrects rounded shoulders and improves posture.

Calf Raises: Rising onto the balls of your feet strengthens the calf muscles, which are essential for maintaining balance and avoiding ankle problems.

4. Frequency and Progress:

Seniors should do muscular activation drills on a regular basis, with at least 2-3 sessions each week.

Begin with light resistance or bodyweight exercises, gradually increasing intensity and complexity as your strength and stability improve.

5. Consultation & Safety:

Before beginning any fitness program, elders should contact a healthcare practitioner or trained trainer to guarantee their safety and appropriateness.

It is critical to listen to your body, prevent overexertion, and alter routines as needed to meet different talents and limits.

Incorporating muscle activation drills into a senior's exercise regimen is critical for injury prevention, stability improvement, and functional independence in everyday tasks.

Seniors can enhance their strength, mobility, and well-being by focusing on important muscle groups and progressively increasing the intensity.

Chapter 4: Strength Training for Functional Fitness

Strength training for functional fitness aims to improve your body's capacity to execute daily tasks effectively and securely.

Unlike traditional bodybuilding, which generally prioritizes aesthetic aims, functional strength training focuses on actions that are similar to real-life activities like lifting groceries, carrying children, or ascending stairs.

Specificity is a basic element of functional strength training. This entails adapting your workouts to replicate the motions you do in ordinary life.

Instead of isolating certain muscles with machines, consider performing complex exercises such as squats, deadlifts, and lunges, which activate many muscle groups at the same time.

Functional strength training stresses core stability and balance. A strong core offers a solid basis for movement and helps to prevent injuries. Planks, bridges, and stability ball exercises are all effective ways to develop core strength and stability.

Functional strength training can improve both everyday chores and athletic performance.

You may increase your agility, power, and endurance by focusing on sports-specific motions. A soccer player, for example, may combine activities that simulate kicking, running, and rapid direction changes.

Another advantage of functional strength training is that it promotes joint health and flexibility. Many functional activities require a broad range of motion, which helps to maintain or enhance joint flexibility. This can increase general mobility while lowering the chance of injury.

When developing a functional strength training program, it is critical to focus on good form and technique.

Improper form during workouts can result in injuries and undermine the advantages of strength training. Begin with lesser weights or resistance bands to learn the exercises before increasing the burden.

Consistency is essential for achieving gains from functional strength training. Aim to add strength training activities into your regimen at least twice to three times per week, with rest days in between to enable your muscles to heal and strengthen.

Functional strength training is an excellent approach to boost your overall fitness and quality of life. Focusing on movements that are applicable to real-world tasks will help you gain strength, stability, and flexibility while lowering your risk of injury. Functional strength exercise, with good technique and consistency, may improve your movement and make you feel stronger in your daily life.

Tailored Resistance Exercises for Older Muscle Groups

Maintaining muscle strength as we age is critical for our general health and independence.

Resistance workouts designed for older muscle groups can help prevent age-related muscle loss (sarcopenia) and enhance functional capacities.

These activities should be safe, effective, and tailored to meet the requirements and limits of older people.

Consultation with a Healthcare Professional: Before beginning any fitness program, older people should check with their doctor to confirm that they may safely participate in resistance training.

This stage is critical for determining any underlying health issues or physical restrictions that may influence the exercise selection process.

Focus on Functional Movements: Tailored workouts should stress functional movements that are similar to regular tasks.

Squats, lunges, step-ups, and overhead presses are some examples of exercises. These motions improve muscular strength, balance, and coordination, resulting in greater mobility and a lower chance of falling.

Progressive resistance training involves gradually increasing resistance over time in order to stimulate muscular development and adaptability.

Older folks can begin with minimal resistance, such as bodyweight exercises or resistance bands, and gradually increase weight as their strength improves. This progressive approach lowers the chance of damage while encouraging continual development.

Target Major Muscle Groups: Resistance exercises should be tailored to specific muscle groups such as the legs, back, chest, shoulders, and arms.

Exercises that activate many muscular groups at once, such as compound movements like squats and deadlifts, improve efficiency and efficacy.

Balance and Stability Exercises: In addition to weight training, balance and stability exercises are vital for preventing falls and improving functional independence.

Exercises that assist older persons retain stability and proprioception include single-leg stands, heel-to-toe walks, and balance board exercises.

Flexibility and Mobility Work: Maintaining flexibility and joint mobility is critical for older persons to conduct everyday tasks comfortably and lower the chance of injury. Stretching exercises that target main muscle groups increase flexibility and range of motion.

Rest and Recovery: Adequate rest and recovery are critical for older people who participate in resistance exercise. Rest days between workouts help muscles heal and get stronger, lowering the chance of overuse problems.

Seniors may maintain or increase their strength, mobility, and independence as they age by following a personalized resistance training program that focuses on functional motions, progressive overload, and general muscle health.

Consulting with a healthcare practitioner and tailoring the program to individual requirements and abilities assures safe and successful outcomes.

Core Stability and Balance Workouts

Core stability and balance workouts are crucial components of any fitness plan since they focus on strengthening core muscles while improving balance and coordination.

These exercises work the muscles in the belly, lower back, hips, and pelvis, establishing a stable foundation for all movement patterns and activities.

Core stability is essential for maintaining good posture, avoiding injuries, and improving sports performance.

It stabilizes the spine, pelvis, and shoulders, ensuring support and alignment throughout daily activities and workouts.

 Core stability also boosts total body control and balance, lowering the chance of falling and improving functional movement patterns.

Balance training enhances proprioception and spatial awareness, in addition to strengthening core muscles. Balance exercises enhance coordination, agility, and response time by activating stabilizing muscles and brain pathways.

Improved balance not only lowers the chance of falling, but it also enhances athletic performance in sports that require fast changes of direction and agility.

Effective Core Stability Exercises:

Front plank, side plank, and reverse plank exercises work the whole core, including the abdominals, obliques, and lower back muscles.

Dead Bug: This exercise works the deep core muscles and improves coordination and stability.

Bird Dog: This exercise improves the back, abdominals, and glutes by testing balance and core stability.

Russian twists are rotational motions that target the obliques and increase core endurance.

Superman: The Superman workout strengthens the lower back and glutes, improving spinal stability and posture.
Effective Balance Exercises:

Single-Leg Balance: Standing on one leg requires proprioception and increases ankle stability.

Bosu Ball Exercises: Squats, lunges, and push-ups on a Bosu ball work core muscles and improve balance and coordination.

Sitting or reclining on a stability ball while completing exercises like crunches or back extensions helps to stimulate core muscles and improve balance.

Yoga and Pilates combine postures and movements to improve balance, flexibility, and core strength via conscious movement and breath control.Incorporating core stability and balance exercises into your training program is critical for general health and performance.

By strengthening core muscles and increasing balance, these exercises improve stability, posture, and functional movement patterns, lowering the risk of injury and boosting athletic performance in a variety of sports.

Integrating Resistance Bands for Added Resistance

Morning workouts provide a refreshing start to the day, particularly for older men who want to preserve their health and vigor.

Integrating resistance bands into these exercises can greatly improve their efficacy by providing additional resistance, resulting in increased strength, balance, and flexibility.

Benefits of resistance bands:

Resistance bands are adaptable, lightweight instruments that provide several benefits for elderly men during morning workouts.

They offer progressive resistance, which means the intensity rises as the band is stretched, providing for a more personalized training experience. Furthermore, resistance bands are easy on the joints, making them perfect for elderly people who may have joint problems or accidents.

Comprehensive Workout Routine:

To effectively use resistance bands into morning exercises, create a complete regimen that targets many muscle areas.

This can include bicep curls, shoulder presses, chest presses, squats, and leg lifts. By combining resistance bands into these exercises, older men may target many muscle groups at once, resulting in a more efficient and effective workout.

Increasing Strength and Muscle Tone:

Resistance bands provide a unique type of resistance that tests muscles in ways that regular weightlifting cannot. Incorporating resistance bands into morning workouts can result in increased strength and muscular tone, allowing older men to maintain their physical independence and mobility as they age.

Improving Balance and Stability:
Maintaining balance and stability is critical for elderly men to avoid falling and injuring themselves.

Resistance bands can be used for workouts that focus on balance and stability, such as standing leg lifts or side leg lifts with the band wrapped around the ankles.

These exercises increase proprioception and strengthen stabilizing muscles, resulting in better overall balance and stability.

Flexible and Range of Motion:

Incorporating resistance bands into morning workouts can also help to increase flexibility and range of motion, which tend to deteriorate as we age.

Dynamic stretching exercises using resistance bands can help older men gain flexibility in important regions including the shoulders, hips, and hamstrings, lowering their risk of injury and improving overall mobility.

Incorporating resistance bands into morning workouts for older men provides a complete and successful approach to improving strength, balance, flexibility, and general physical health.

By including these adaptable tools into their regimens, older men may get the advantages of a well-rounded workout that promotes long-term health and vitality.

Chapter 5: Cardiovascular Conditioning for Longevity

As men age, preserving cardiovascular health becomes increasingly important for their lifespan and general well-being.

A morning training practice designed exclusively for elderly men can considerably improve cardiovascular fitness, endurance, heart health, and lifespan. Here's a complete guide to a morning workout regimen aimed at improving cardiovascular fitness.

Warm-Up (5 minutes): Begin with a simple warm-up to get the body ready for workout. This might involve brisk walking, mild running in place, or dynamic stretches to relax muscles and improve blood flow.

Cardiovascular Exercise (20-30 minutes): Perform moderate-intensity cardiovascular exercises such brisk walking, cycling, swimming, or utilizing a stationary bike or elliptical machine.

Aim for at least 20-30 minutes of continuous movement to increase heart rate and cardiovascular endurance.

Interval Training (10 minutes): Use interval training to test the cardiovascular system and increase metabolism. Alternate between higher effort (e.g., quicker walking or cycling) and lower intensity (e.g., slower pace or active recovery) for 1-2 minute intervals.

Strength Training (15-20 minutes): Perform strength training exercises to maintain muscle mass, promote joint health, and improve total functional fitness. Focus on complex exercises that target key muscular groups, such as bodyweight squats, lunges, push-ups, and seated rows with resistance bands or modest weights.

Cool Down and Stretching (5-10 minutes): After the workout, take a cooldown period to gradually drop your heart rate and avoid dizziness or pain.

To enhance flexibility and reduce muscular tension, perform static stretches that target key muscle groups. Hold each stretch for 15-30 seconds.

Hydration and Nutrition: Drinking water or electrolyte-rich drinks will keep you hydrated during your workout. To boost recovery and fuel energy levels, follow your workout with a balanced breakfast that includes lean protein, healthy fats, complex carbs, and lots of fruits and vegetables.

Consistency and Progression: Repeat this morning workout regimen at least 3-5 times each week, progressively increasing the intensity or duration as fitness improves. Listen to your body, adapt your workout intensity as needed, and speak with a healthcare expert before beginning any new fitness program, especially if you are older or have pre-existing health concerns.

Older men can improve their health, increase their lifespan, and live a better life by putting cardiovascular conditioning first in an organized morning workout regimen.

Endurance-Boosting Cardiovascular Workouts

Endurance-boosting cardiovascular activities are critical for preserving overall health and energy, particularly as we age.

Incorporating morning workouts into older men's routines can have various benefits, including improved cardiovascular health, greater energy levels, and improved mental clarity throughout the day.

Here are some thorough and simple morning routines designed exclusively for elderly guys to improve endurance:

Brisk walking is a basic but efficient morning workout that gets the heart rate up and the blood flowing without placing too much strain on the joints. Older men can begin at a modest pace, gradually increasing speed and length as their endurance increases.

For maximum cardiovascular advantages, aim for at least 30 minutes of brisk walking.

Cycling: Cycling is a low-impact sport that provides an excellent cardiovascular workout for elderly men.

Cycling, whether on a stationary bike or outside, strengthens the heart and lungs while training the leg muscles. For extra encouragement, older men can go for a morning bike ride around their neighborhood or explore picturesque routes.

Swimming is a great alternative for elderly men who want a full-body workout that is easy on their joints. Swimming works numerous muscle groups and provides cardiovascular strain.

Morning swims in a pool or natural body of water may wake up the body and mind, establishing a good tone for the day ahead.

Elliptical machines are a low-impact alternative to classic cardio activities such as running and jogging.

Elliptical exercise can help older men build endurance, burn calories, and develop their upper and lower body muscles. Begin with a comfortable resistance level and progressively raise the intensity as fitness improves.

Stair Climbing: Climbing steps is an easy and efficient approach for elderly men to improve their cardiovascular endurance while also improving lower body strength. Stair climbing, whether done on a stair climber machine or outdoors, works the heart, lungs, and leg muscles for a full-body morning exercise.

Incorporating these endurance-boosting cardiovascular activities into a morning regimen can help older men improve their overall fitness, enhance their energy levels, and stay in good health as they age. Remember to see a healthcare expert before beginning any new fitness regimen, especially if you have pre-existing health concerns.

High-Intensity Interval Training (HIIT) for Older Men

High-Intensity Interval Training (HIIT) has been popular in recent years due to its effectiveness in increasing cardiovascular health, muscle strength, and general fitness.

While HIIT is commonly associated with younger people, it may also be quite useful for older men, providing a time-saving and effective fitness schedule suited to their specific requirements and skills.

Benefits for Older Men: High-intensity interval training (HIIT) can improve cardiovascular health, muscular mass, metabolism, and overall fitness levels.

According to research, HIIT can be especially helpful in improving cardiovascular function and reversing age-related muscle mass and strength loss.

Safety Considerations: Before beginning a high-intensity interval training program, older men should check with their healthcare physician, especially if they have any pre-existing medical illnesses or concerns.

To minimize injury and overexertion, HIIT programs should begin cautiously and progressively build in intensity and length.

Tailoring exercises: HIIT exercises may be simply adapted to older men's fitness levels and skills. Exercises can be adapted to have lower-impact versions, and rest times can be varied to ensure proper recovery.

Using a range of exercises that target different muscle groups can help prevent overuse problems and keep workouts interesting.

A example HIIT program for older men may comprise a warm-up phase of 5-10 minutes of gentle cardiovascular activity, followed by a series of high-intensity intervals (e.g., 30 seconds of hard exercise followed by 60 seconds of rest) lasting 20-30 minutes.

Squats, lunges, push-ups, and jumping jacks are examples of bodyweight workouts, as are cardio exercises like cycling or swimming.

Progression and Adaptation: As older men grow more used to HIIT, they may progressively raise the intensity and duration of their workouts to keep challenging their bodies and improving their fitness levels.

To avoid burnout or injury, athletes must listen to their bodies and alter their training accordingly.

High-Intensity Interval Training (HIIT) may be a very effective and efficient training plan for older men, providing several health advantages while also improving overall fitness levels. With appropriate supervision and changes, older men may safely adopt HIIT into their training routines, allowing them to remain healthy, active, and powerful.

Incorporating Low-Impact Aerobics
for Joint Health

Incorporating low-impact aerobics into your morning workout program is a wise decision, particularly for older men worried about joint health.

Low-impact aerobics provide several advantages while putting less strain on joints, making them an excellent type of exercise for preserving joint health and general fitness.

Low-impact aerobics includes joint-friendly exercises including walking, swimming, cycling, and utilizing elliptical machines.

These workouts increase cardiovascular health, flexibility, and muscular strength while minimizing joint stress.

One of the key benefits of low-impact aerobics is that they lessen the likelihood of joint injury.

Unlike high-impact workouts like running or leaping, which may put a strain on the knees, hips, and ankles, low-impact aerobics are a safer option that reduces the chance of joint pain and injury.

Using low-impact aerobics in your early workout program helps increase joint mobility and flexibility.

Regular movement lubricates the joints and increases the circulation of synovial fluid, which nourishes and protects the cartilage.

This can result in greater range of motion and decreased stiffness, making daily tasks simpler and more pleasant.Low-impact exercises also help with weight management.

Excess weight can worsen joint discomfort and inflammation, especially in weight-bearing joints such as the knees and hips. Older men can maintain a healthy weight by engaging in regular aerobic activity, which reduces joint strain and alleviates discomfort.

Low-impact aerobics can improve both physical and mental health. Exercise causes the production of endorphins, chemicals that increase happiness and relieve stress. Starting your day with a morning workout can improve your attitude and energy levels, establishing a good tone for the remainder of the day.

To add low-impact aerobics into your daily routine, begin with a quick warm-up to prepare your muscles and joints for activity. Choose activities that you love and are comfortable with, then gradually increase the time and intensity as your fitness improves. Remember to listen to your body and alter activities as necessary to avoid discomfort or damage.

Overall, incorporating low-impact aerobics into your morning workout regimen may be extremely helpful to joint health, providing a safe and effective approach to remain active and fit as you get older.

Chapter 6: Recovery and Regeneration Strategies

Recovery and regeneration tactics are critical components of every good training program, regardless of the individual objectives or sports activities.

These tactics seek to maximize the body's ability to recover from physical activity, reduce the chance of injury, and improve overall performance. Here are some of the major components of recovery and regeneration strategies:

Rest and Sleep: Adequate rest and quality sleep are critical to healing. During sleep, the body goes through important restorative processes include muscular development and repair, hormone balance, and mental refreshment.

Aim for 7-9 hours of unbroken sleep every night to promote healthy recuperation.

Nutrition: Proper nutrition is essential for healing and regeneration. A well-balanced diet rich in lean proteins, complex carbs, healthy fats, vitamins, and minerals provides the body with the nutrition it needs to repair tissues, refill glycogen reserves, and promote general recovery.

Hydration: Hydration is essential for several physiological activities, including nutrition delivery, temperature control, and waste disposal.
  Drink plenty of water throughout the day, and consider using electrolyte-rich drinks to restore minerals lost during strenuous activities.

Active Recovery: Light, low-impact exercises like walking, cycling, or swimming can increase blood flow, improve nutrition supply to muscles, and help in the elimination of metabolic waste products. Incorporate active recovery exercises into your training plan to improve overall recovery while without overtaxing the body.

Stretching and Mobility: Including stretching exercises and mobility drills in your workout program will help you increase your flexibility, range of motion, and muscle elasticity.

Stretching increases blood flow to muscles, decreases muscular tension, and avoids stiffness, which improves recovery and lowers the chance of injury.

Massage treatment and foam rolling are both efficient procedures for relieving muscular tension, breaking up scar tissue, and increasing blood circulation.

Regular massage or self-myofascial release using foam rollers can help relieve muscular stiffness and improve recovery after strenuous activities.

Mind-Body Techniques: Meditation, deep breathing exercises, and relaxation techniques can help decrease stress, improve mental clarity, and general well-being. Incorporating mind-body methods into your daily routine can aid in overall recovery and regeneration.

Periodization: By structuring your training program with high intensity intervals followed by low intensity or active rest times, you may ensure appropriate recovery and adaptability.

Implementing a well-designed periodization plan gives your body enough time to recuperate and adjust to training stimuli, resulting in long-term performance gains.

By implementing these recovery and regeneration tactics into your training plan, you may improve your body's ability to recover from physical activity, reduce the chance of injury, and ultimately improve your overall performance and well-being.

Importance of Post-Workout Nutrition for Muscle Repair

Morning workouts for older men may be a great way to start the day and enhance their general health. However, the value of post-workout nutrition cannot be overemphasized, particularly in terms of muscle regeneration and recovery.

As we age, our bodies go through physiological changes that might affect muscle repair and development.

As a result, older men who exercise in the morning must pay special attention to their post-workout diet in order to maximize muscle recovery and general health.

1. *Protein Intake:* Protein is required for muscle repair and development. Following a morning workout, older men should have a protein-rich breakfast or snack to give their muscles the building blocks needed for restoration. Aim for a variety of high-quality protein sources, including lean meats, eggs, dairy products, and plant-based alternatives like beans and lentils.

2. *Carbohydrate Replenishment:* Carbohydrates replenish glycogen reserves, the major fuel source for activity. To replenish energy and aid in muscle regeneration, older men should include

complex carbs in their post-workout meal. Choose whole grains, fruits, and vegetables to provide a consistent flow of energy throughout the day.

3. *Hydration:* Remaining hydrated is crucial for good health and muscular performance. After a morning workout, older men should restore fluids lost via perspiration by drinking water or electrolyte-rich drinks.

Proper hydration promotes nutrition delivery to muscles and the elimination of metabolic waste products.

4. Nutrient Timing: Optimal post-workout nutrition is critical for muscle repair and recovery. Consuming a balanced breakfast or snack 30 minutes to an hour after exercise will boost protein synthesis and glycogen resynthesis, resulting in speedier recovery and adaptability to training.

5. Anti-inflammatory Foods: Including anti-inflammatory foods in post-workout nutrition helps lessen muscular pain and inflammation, especially for elderly men who may have slower recovery.

Include meals high in omega-3 fatty acids, such as fatty fish, nuts, and seeds, as well as colorful fruits and vegetables high in antioxidants.

Post-workout nutrition is critical for muscle regeneration and recovery, particularly for older men who work out in the mornings.

By focusing on protein consumption, carbohydrate replenishment, hydration, nutritional timing, and anti-inflammatory foods, older men can improve their exercise performance, increase muscle building, and improve their general health and well-being.

Flexibility and Mobility Routines for
Enhanced Recovery

Morning workouts for older men may be both energizing and useful to their general health, but integrating flexibility and mobility routines is critical for improving recovery and avoiding injury.

These exercises aim to improve range of motion, reduce stiffness, and promote better movement patterns. This is a complete approach to incorporating flexibility and mobility practices into morning workouts for older men.

1. Begin with an active warm-up to stimulate blood flow and prepare the body for exercise. This may involve arm circles, leg swings, hip circles, and shoulder rotations.

2. *Foam Rolling:* Use foam rolling to alleviate muscular tension and increase tissue quality. Concentrate on regions prone to tension, such as the calves, hamstrings, quadriceps, gluteus, and upper back.

3. *Stretching:* Perform static stretches for main muscle groups. Focus on the hamstrings, quadriceps, calves, chest, shoulders, and back. Hold each stretch for 15-30 seconds, aiming for a mild stretch with no discomfort.

4. *Mobility Exercises:* Incorporate mobility exercises to enhance joint function and movement quality. Hip circles, shoulder dislocates, thoracic rotations, and ankle mobility workouts can all help you improve your overall mobility.

5. *Consider including yoga or Pilates into your morning regimen*. These exercises emphasize flexibility, balance, and core strength, all of which are necessary for older men to stay mobile and avoid accidents.

6. *Balance Training:* Use balance exercises to increase stability and lessen the danger of falling. Simple activities that increase balance and proprioception include single-leg stands, heel-to-toe walks, and standing on a balance board.

7. *Cool Down:* After your workout, take a good cool down to help with recuperation. Gentle stretching, deep breathing exercises, and relaxation techniques can all help to relax the muscles and reduce stress.

8. *Consistency:* Consistency is essential for seeing outcomes. Incorporating flexibility and mobility practices into your morning workouts on a regular basis will provide long-term advantages.

By including these flexibility and mobility routines into morning workouts, older men may increase recovery, improve movement quality, and lower their risk of injury, resulting in a healthier and more active lifestyle.

Remember to listen to your body and change workouts as necessary to meet your specific requirements and abilities.

Mindfulness Techniques for Stress Reduction and Sleep Improvement

In today's fast-paced world, stress has become an unavoidable aspect of existence, frequently resulting in sleep problems and general poor well-being. Incorporating mindfulness practices into your everyday routine can help you manage stress and get better sleep.

Here are some extensive and simple mindfulness exercises for stress reduction and sleep enhancement.

attentive breathing: Begin each day with a few minutes of attentive breathing.

Concentrate on how you breath by closing your eyes and comfortably lie down

Feel the sensation of air entering and exiting your body. This easy exercise can help you relax, reduce tension, and prepare for a good night's sleep.

Body Scan Meditation: Take a few minutes to practice body scan meditation. Close your eyes and focus your attention on different regions of your body, beginning with your toes and gradually progressing to your head.

Recognize any tension or pain and intentionally relax those regions. This exercise encourages relaxation and relieves physical stress, resulting in better sleep.

Mindful Eating: Practice mindful eating throughout the day by focusing on the sensory experience of eating. Consider the colors, textures, tastes, and aromas of your meal.

Chew gently and relish every bite. Eating mindfully can help reduce stress by instilling a sense of presence and fulfillment, which can improve sleep quality.

Gratitude Journaling: Before going to bed, take a few minutes to jot down three things you are grateful for each day.

Focusing on the good things in your life may change your mentality from stress to thankfulness, encouraging feelings of happiness and well-being. This practice can help you relax and sleep better by instilling a sense of serenity and happiness.

Progressive Muscle Relaxation: Add progressive muscle relaxation to your sleep regimen. Begin by tensing and carefully releasing each muscle group in your body, beginning with your toes and progressing up to your head.

This exercise relieves physical stress and promotes relaxation, making it easier to fall and remain asleep during the night.

By implementing these mindfulness practices into your daily routine, you may successfully reduce stress and enhance the quality of your sleep, resulting in increased overall well-being and vitality.

Now, let's look at an excellent morning workout regimen made exclusively for senior guys.

Chapter 7: Tailoring Your Morning Workout Routine

Creating a customized morning fitness regimen for older men is critical for maintaining general health, strength, and flexibility. Here's a detailed guide to help you create an effective and efficient training routine:

Warm-Up: Start your daily routine with a mild warm-up to improve blood flow and prepare your muscles for a workout. This can involve 5–10 minutes of light cardio, such as walking or cycling, followed by dynamic stretches to relax joints and increase flexibility.

Strength Training: Use resistance workouts that target key muscle groups to increase strength and bone density. Concentrate on compound exercises such as squats, lunges, chest presses, rows, and overhead presses using dumbbells, resistance bands, or bodyweight. Aim for 2-3 sets of 8-12 repetitions every exercise, with excellent form and controlled movement.

Balance and Stability: As we age, keeping balance and stability becomes increasingly vital in avoiding falls and accidents. Balance exercises such as single-leg stands, heel-to-toe walks, and stability ball exercises will help you improve your coordination and core strength.

Stretching activities can help you increase your flexibility and mobility. Perform static stretches that target key muscle groups, holding each stretch for 15 to 30 seconds without bouncing. Concentrate on regions prone to stiffness such as the hips, hamstrings, shoulders, and low back.

Cardiovascular Exercise: Engage in cardiovascular exercises to improve your heart health and endurance. Choose low-impact activities such as brisk walking, swimming, cycling, or utilizing an elliptical machine to reduce joint strain while increasing heart rate.

Aim for at least 20-30 minutes of moderate-intensity cardio, progressively increasing the length and intensity as fitness improves.

Cool down and stretch: After your workout, take a cooldown period to gradually drop your heart rate and avoid muscular discomfort. Gently stretch the muscles used throughout your workout, holding each stretch for 15-30 seconds to improve relaxation and flexibility.

Hydration and Nutrition: Stay hydrated during your workout and replace electrolytes lost via sweating. Consume a well-balanced post-workout breakfast or snack high in protein and carbs to aid muscle repair and restore energy storage.

Rest and Recovery: Allow enough time between workout sessions to avoid overtraining and encourage muscle regeneration. Allow at least 48 hours of recuperation before addressing the same muscle groups again.

By adapting your morning training regimen to the special demands of older men, you may increase overall fitness, improve quality of life, and age gracefully while remaining vital and strong.

Creating a Personalized Workout Plan for Older Men

Developing a specific training regimen for older men is critical for preserving physical health, increasing mobility, and avoiding age-related diseases.

As men age, their bodies suffer a variety of changes, including muscle loss, lower bone density, and less flexibility. A personalized fitness plan can help address these difficulties and boost general health.

First and foremost, before beginning any new exercise program, speak with a healthcare practitioner, especially for older persons with pre-existing medical issues or

mobility constraints.
Once cleared, the fitness routine should include a mix of strength training, aerobic activity, flexibility, and balancing activities.

Strength training is especially crucial for elderly men to prevent muscle loss and preserve bone density. It should contain workouts that target key muscular areas including squats,

lunges, chest presses, rows, and bicep curls. Resistance bands, free weights, or weight machines can be employed depending on personal preferences and skills.

Cardiovascular exercise promotes heart health and endurance. Older folks benefit from activities such as brisk walking, cycling, swimming, and low-impact aerobics. Begin with shorter workouts and progressively increase the time and intensity as fitness improves.

Flexibility exercises are vital for preserving range of motion and avoiding injury. Stretching exercises should target all main muscle groups and be done following a warm-up or at the end of a workout. Yoga and tai chi are great ways to improve flexibility, balance, and relaxation.

Balance exercises are important for preventing falls, which are a significant worry among older persons. Balance and coordination may be improved with simple exercises such as standing on one leg, heel-to-toe walking, or utilizing stability.

Integrating rest days into the workout schedule is critical for enabling the body to recuperate and avoiding overtraining. Individual development, preferences, and any health problems that occur should all be taken into account when making plan adjustments.

Consistency is essential while following a specific fitness regimen. Regular exercise, when paired with correct diet and adequate rest, may dramatically enhance the quality of life for older men, allowing them to remain active, independent, and healthy as they age.

Adaptations for Individual Needs and Limitations

Morning workouts for elderly men include adapting routines to their specific demands and restrictions. It is critical to prioritize low-impact exercises that improve strength, flexibility, and cardiovascular health while reducing the chance of injury.

Warm-up activities are necessary to prepare the body for physical activity. Gentle motions like arm circles, shoulder rolls, and walking in place improve blood flow to muscles and joints, lowering the incidence of strains and sprains.

Walking or cycling at a moderate speed is beneficial to cardiovascular health. These activities give a low-impact technique to increase heart rate without placing undue strain on joints. Swimming and water aerobics are other good possibilities since water's buoyancy decreases joint impact.

Strength training is vital for preserving muscle mass and bone density, both of which tend to deteriorate as we age.

However, it is critical to select workouts suited for older persons. Bodyweight exercises like squats, lunges, and modified push-ups can help improve strength without the need of heavy equipment.

Flexibility exercises are critical for preserving range of motion and avoiding stiffness. Gentle stretches for key muscle groups, such as the shoulders, back, hips, and legs, can be included in your training program.

Yoga or tai chi programs created exclusively for elders can also help improve flexibility and balance.

Balance exercises are especially helpful for elderly persons to lower their risk of falling. Standing on one leg, walking heel-to-toe, or utilizing a balancing board can all help you improve your stability and coordination.

It's critical to listen to your body and make changes as required. Older men may require longer rest periods between exercises or lower the intensity of specific motions.

Encouraging kids to keep hydrated and heed to their body' signs is critical for avoiding overexertion.

Cool-down stretches and relaxation exercises are critical for improving healing and reducing muscular discomfort. Gentle stretching and deep breathing exercises can reduce heart rate and improve calm.

By tailoring early exercises to their specific requirements and limits, older men may get the advantages of regular physical activity while reducing the risk of injury and pain. With an emphasis on low-impact workouts that build strength, flexibility, cardiovascular health, and balance, older persons can have a healthy and active lifestyle for many years.

Tracking Progress and Adjusting Goals for Sustainable Results

Morning workouts for older men are critical to preserving physical health, vigor, and general well-being. To guarantee long-term success on this fitness journey, it is critical to employ appropriate tracking systems and change goals as needed.

1. Set clear objectives: Before beginning a morning training plan, elderly men should create clear fitness goals. Setting precise goals, whether for cardiovascular health, strength and flexibility, or weight management, gives direction and incentive.

2. Use Tracking Tools: Tracking progress is critical for determining the efficacy of a morning training routine. Older men can use exercise apps, wearable devices, or basic journaling to log workouts, track performance metrics, and track progress over time.

3. *Track Physical Changes:* Progress is more than just putting numbers on a scale and lifting greater weights. It's also about noting tiny bodily improvements like higher energy, greater mobility, and better posture. Paying attention to these changes might provide hopeful indicators of growth.

4. *Regular Assessments:* Periodic evaluations are essential for determining progress and finding areas for improvement. Older men can undergo frequent fitness exams to analyze body composition, flexibility, endurance, and strength, allowing them to tailor their training programs accordingly.

5. *Adjust Goals Wisely:* As fitness levels increase, goals may need to be altered to keep momentum and avoid plateauing. To advance in their morning exercises, older men should review their aims on a regular basis and create new, tough but doable goals.

6. *Listen to Your Body:* Older bodies have different requirements and limits than younger ones. It is critical for older men to listen to their bodies, detect signals of weariness or injury, and adapt training intensity or length accordingly to avoid overexertion and ensure long-term endurance.

7. *Seek Professional Advice:* Consulting with fitness professionals or healthcare providers can give significant insights and tailored advice for improving morning training regimens.

Professionals may provide personalized fitness routines, dietary recommendations, and injury prevention measures based on individual requirements and objectives.

Tracking progress and changing objectives are critical components of long-term outcomes in morning workouts for older men.

Older men may reach and maintain optimal fitness levels for enhanced health and well-being by setting clear goals, using tracking tools, monitoring physical changes, doing regular assessments, modifying goals strategically, listening to their bodies, and seeking expert advice.

CONCLUSION

Morning workouts have various benefits for older men, including improved physical and mental health and addressing age-related problems.

Exercise in the morning boosts metabolism, aids with weight control, and lowers the risk of chronic disorders like diabetes and heart disease. Morning exercises can help men regain mental sharpness and emotional equilibrium as they age.

Exercising in the morning sets a good tone for the day, increasing productivity and general energy levels. For older men, this can be especially effective in combating age-related weariness and maintaining an active lifestyle.

Furthermore, morning workouts allow for social engagement, whether through group sessions or outdoor activities, which promotes a sense of camaraderie and support among peers.

However, older men should pursue early activities with caution, taking into account their own fitness levels and any pre-existing health concerns.

Consulting a healthcare practitioner and working with a trained fitness instructor can assist older men in developing a safe and successful training plan.

Overall, including morning workouts into one's daily routine can considerably improve the quality of life for older men, boosting longevity and vitality in their golden years.

THANK YOU PAGE

Thank you for selecting this book. Your support is really appreciated. Similarly, I am grateful for the purchase of this book.

Your input is valuable; please share your ideas in a review. It serves as a reference for future improvements. Enjoy reading and utilizing it!

Weekly
Workout Planner

Week :_____________

Month: _____________

Sunday

Monday

Tuesday

Goals

Goals

Goals

Wednesday

Thursday

Friday

Goals

Goals

Goals

Saturday

Water Tracker

Goals

Mood

Motivation ________________________________

Weekly
Workout Planner

Week : _______________

Month: _______________

Sunday

Monday

Tuesday

Goals

Goals

Goals

Wednesday

Thursday

Friday

Goals

Goals

Goals

Saturday

Water Tracker

Goals

Mood

Motivation _______________________________

Weekly
Workout Planner

Week : ___________

Month: ___________

Sunday	Monday	Tuesday
Goals	Goals	Goals

Wednesday	Thursday	Friday
Goals	Goals	Goals

Saturday

Water Tracker

Goals

Mood

Motivation ________________________________
____
____
____
____

Weekly
Workout Planner

Week :________________

Month:________________

Sunday

Monday

Tuesday

Goals

Goals

Goals

Wednesday

Thursday

Friday

Goals

Goals

Goals

Saturday

Water Tracker

Goals

Mood

Motivation ________________________________

Weekly
Workout Planner

Week : _______________

Month: _______________

Sunday	Monday	Tuesday
Goals	Goals	Goals

Wednesday	Thursday	Friday
Goals	Goals	Goals

Saturday

Goals

Water Tracker

Mood

Motivation ________________________

____

____

____

____

____

Weekly
Workout Planner

Week : _______________

Month: _______________

Sunday	Monday	Tuesday
Goals	Goals	Goals

Wednesday	Thursday	Friday
Goals	Goals	Goals

Saturday

Goals

Water Tracker

Mood

Motivation ________________________________

____

____

____

____

Weekly
Workout Planner

Week :________________

Month: ________________

Sunday	Monday	Tuesday
Goals	Goals	Goals

Wednesday	Thursday	Friday
Goals	Goals	Goals

Saturday

Goals

Water Tracker

Mood

Goals

Motivation ____________________
____
____
____
____

Weekly
Workout Planner

Week : _______________

Month: _______________

Sunday

Monday

Tuesday

Goals

Goals

Goals

Wednesday

Thursday

Friday

Goals

Goals

Goals

Saturday

Water Tracker

Goals

Mood

Motivation ____

____

____

____

____

Weekly
Workout Planner

Week : ___________

Month: ___________

Sunday

Monday

Tuesday

Goals

Goals

Goals

Wednesday

Thursday

Friday

Goals

Goals

Goals

Saturday

Water Tracker

Goals

Mood

Motivation ____________________

Weekly
Workout Planner

Week : _______________

Month: _______________

Sunday	Monday	Tuesday
Goals	Goals	Goals

Wednesday	Thursday	Friday
Goals	Goals	Goals

Saturday

Goals

Water Tracker

Mood

Motivation _______________________________________
____
____
____
____

Weekly
Workout Planner

Week: ___________

Month: ___________

Sunday	Monday	Tuesday
Goals	Goals	Goals

Wednesday	Thursday	Friday
Goals	Goals	Goals

Saturday

Goals

Water Tracker

Mood

Motivation ____

____

____

____

____

Weekly
Workout Planner

Week : _______________

Month: _______________

Sunday

Monday

Tuesday

Goals

Goals

Goals

Wednesday

Thursday

Friday

Goals

Goals

Goals

Saturday

Water Tracker

Goals

Mood

Motivation ____

Weekly
Workout Planner

Week : __________

Month: __________

Sunday	Monday	Tuesday

Goals · Goals · Goals

Wednesday	Thursday	Friday

Goals · Goals · Goals

Saturday

Water Tracker

Goals

Mood

Motivation _______________________________

Weekly
Workout Planner

Week : _______________

Month: _______________

Sunday   Monday   Tuesday

Goals   Goals   Goals

Wednesday   Thursday   Friday

Goals   Goals   Goals

Saturday   Water Tracker

Goals   Mood

Motivation _______________________________

Weekly
Workout Planner

Week :________________

Month: ________________

Sunday   Monday   Tuesday

Goals   Goals   Goals

Wednesday   Thursday   Friday

Goals   Goals   Goals

Saturday   Water Tracker

Goals   Mood

Motivation ____
____
____
____
____
____

Weekly
Workout Planner

Week : _______________

Month: _______________

Sunday   Monday   Tuesday

Goals   Goals   Goals

Wednesday   Thursday   Friday

Goals   Goals   Goals

Saturday   Water Tracker

Goals   Mood

Motivation ____
____
____
____
____

Weekly
Workout Planner

Week :_____________

Month:_____________

Sunday	Monday	Tuesday
Goals	Goals	Goals

Wednesday	Thursday	Friday
Goals	Goals	Goals

Saturday

Water Tracker

Goals

Mood

Motivation ___________________________
____
____
____
____

Weekly
Workout Planner

Week : ______________

Month: ______________

Sunday

Monday

Tuesday

Goals

Goals

Goals

Wednesday

Thursday

Friday

Goals

Goals

Goals

Saturday

Water Tracker

Goals

Mood

Motivation ________________________________

____

____

____

____

Weekly
Workout Planner

Week : ___________

Month: ___________

Sunday	Monday	Tuesday
Goals	Goals	Goals

Wednesday	Thursday	Friday
Goals	Goals	Goals

Saturday

Goals

Water Tracker

Mood

Motivation ________________________________

____

____

____

____

Weekly
Workout Planner

Week :____________

Month:____________

Sunday

Monday

Tuesday

Goals

Goals

Goals

Wednesday

Thursday

Friday

Goals

Goals

Goals

Saturday

Water Tracker

Goals

Mood

Motivation

Weekly
Workout Planner

Week : ______________

Month: ______________

Sunday

Monday

Tuesday

Goals

Goals

Goals

Wednesday

Thursday

Friday

Goals

Goals

Goals

Saturday

Water Tracker

Goals

Mood

Motivation ________________________________

Weekly
Workout Planner

Week : _______________

Month: _______________

Sunday

Monday

Tuesday

Goals

Goals

Goals

Wednesday

Thursday

Friday

Goals

Goals

Goals

Saturday

Water Tracker

Goals

Mood

Motivation ____

____

____

____

____

Weekly
Workout Planner

Week :____________

Month:____________

Sunday

Monday

Tuesday

Goals

Goals

Goals

Wednesday

Thursday

Friday

Goals

Goals

Goals

Saturday

Water Tracker

Goals

Mood

Motivation ________________________________

Weekly
Workout Planner

Week : _______________

Month: _______________

Sunday   Monday   Tuesday

Goals   Goals   Goals

Wednesday   Thursday   Friday

Goals   Goals   Goals

Saturday   Water Tracker

Goals   Mood

Motivation _______________________

Weekly
Workout Planner

Week :__________

Month:__________

Sunday

Monday

Tuesday

Goals

Goals

Goals

Wednesday

Thursday

Friday

Goals

Goals

Goals

Saturday

Water Tracker

Goals

Mood

Motivation

Weekly
Workout Planner

Week : ________________

Month: ________________

Sunday	Monday	Tuesday
Goals	Goals	Goals

Wednesday	Thursday	Friday
Goals	Goals	Goals

Saturday

Goals

Water Tracker

Mood

Motivation ________________

Weekly
Workout Planner

Week : _______________

Month: _______________

Sunday   Monday   Tuesday

Goals   Goals   Goals

Wednesday   Thursday   Friday

Goals   Goals   Goals

Saturday   Water Tracker

Goals   Mood

Motivation ____________________________

Weekly
Workout Planner

Week : __________________

Month: ________________

Sunday	Monday	Tuesday
Goals	Goals	Goals

Wednesday	Thursday	Friday
Goals	Goals	Goals

Saturday

Goals

Water Tracker

Mood

Motivation ____

Weekly
Workout Planner

Week : __________

Month: __________

Sunday	Monday	Tuesday
Goals	Goals	Goals

Wednesday	Thursday	Friday
Goals	Goals	Goals

Saturday

Goals

Water Tracker

Mood

Motivation ____
____
____
____
____

Weekly
Workout Planner

Week :______________

Month:______________

Sunday

Monday

Tuesday

Goals

Goals

Goals

Wednesday

Thursday

Friday

Goals

Goals

Goals

Saturday

Water Tracker

Goals

Mood

Motivation _______________________________________

Weekly
Workout Planner

Week :_______________

Month: _______________

Sunday	Monday	Tuesday
Goals	Goals	Goals

Wednesday	Thursday	Friday
Goals	Goals	Goals

Saturday

Goals

Water Tracker

Mood

Motivation ___________________________

Weekly
Workout Planner

Week : _______________

Month: _______________

Sunday

Monday

Tuesday

Goals

Goals

Goals

Wednesday

Thursday

Friday

Goals

Goals

Goals

Saturday

Water Tracker

Goals

Mood

Motivation _______________________________________

____

____

____

____

Weekly

Workout Planner

Week : _____________

Month: _____________

Sunday	Monday	Tuesday
Goals	Goals	Goals

Wednesday	Thursday	Friday
Goals	Goals	Goals

Saturday

Goals

Water Tracker

Mood

Motivation ___________________________

Weekly
Workout Planner

Week : _______________

Month: _______________

Sunday

Monday

Tuesday

Goals

Goals

Goals

Wednesday

Thursday

Friday

Goals

Goals

Goals

Saturday

Water Tracker

Goals

Mood

Motivation _______________________________________

Weekly
Workout Planner

Week : _____________

Month: _____________

Sunday	Monday	Tuesday
Goals	Goals	Goals

Wednesday	Thursday	Friday
Goals	Goals	Goals

Saturday

Goals

Water Tracker

Mood

Motivation ________________________________

____

____

____

____

Weekly
Workout Planner

Week : __________________

Month: __________________

Sunday

Monday

Tuesday

Goals

Goals

Goals

Wednesday

Thursday

Friday

Goals

Goals

Goals

Saturday

Water Tracker

Goals

Mood

Motivation ____________________________________
____
____
____
____

Weekly Workout Planner

Week :______________

Month: ______________

Sunday	Monday	Tuesday
Goals	Goals	Goals

Wednesday	Thursday	Friday
Goals	Goals	Goals

Saturday

Goals

Water Tracker

Mood

Motivation ________________

Weekly
Workout Planner

Week : _______________

Month: _______________

Sunday	Monday	Tuesday
Goals	Goals	Goals

Wednesday	Thursday	Friday
Goals	Goals	Goals

Saturday

Goals

Water Tracker

Mood

Motivation __________________________

____

____

____

____

Weekly
Workout Planner

Week :________________

Month:________________

Sunday	Monday	Tuesday
Goals	Goals	Goals

Wednesday	Thursday	Friday
Goals	Goals	Goals

Saturday

Goals

Water Tracker

Mood

Motivation ________________________________

____

____

____

____

Weekly
Workout Planner

Week :___________

Month: ___________

Sunday	Monday	Tuesday
Goals	Goals	Goals

Wednesday	Thursday	Friday
Goals	Goals	Goals

Saturday	Water Tracker
Goals	Mood

Motivation

Weekly
Workout Planner

Week :____________

Month: ____________

Sunday

Monday

Tuesday

Goals

Goals

Goals

Wednesday

Thursday

Friday

Goals

Goals

Goals

Saturday

Water Tracker

Goals

Mood

Motivation ________________________________
____
____
____
____

Weekly
Workout Planner

Week : _______________

Month: _______________

Sunday

Monday

Tuesday

Goals

Goals

Goals

Wednesday

Thursday

Friday

Goals

Goals

Goals

Saturday

Water Tracker

Goals

Mood

Motivation

Weekly
Workout Planner

Week :________________

Month: ________________

Sunday	Monday	Tuesday
Goals	Goals	Goals

Wednesday	Thursday	Friday
Goals	Goals	Goals

Saturday

Goals

Water Tracker

Mood

Motivation ________________

____

____

____

____

Weekly
Workout Planner

Week : _______________

Month: _______________

Sunday   Monday   Tuesday

Goals   Goals   Goals

Wednesday   Thursday   Friday

Goals   Goals   Goals

Saturday   Water Tracker

Goals   Mood

Motivation _______________

Weekly
Workout Planner

Week :______________

Month: ______________

Sunday

Monday

Tuesday

Goals

Goals

Goals

Wednesday

Thursday

Friday

Goals

Goals

Goals

Saturday

Water Tracker

Goals

Mood

Motivation ______________________________

Weekly
Workout Planner

Week : __________

Month: __________

Sunday   Monday   Tuesday

Goals   Goals   Goals

Wednesday   Thursday   Friday

Goals   Goals   Goals

Saturday

Water Tracker

Goals

Mood

Motivation

Weekly
Workout Planner

Week :______________

Month:______________

Sunday

Monday

Tuesday

Goals

Goals

Goals

Wednesday

Thursday

Friday

Goals

Goals

Goals

Saturday

Water Tracker

Goals

Mood

Motivation ____________________________
____
____
____
____

Weekly
Workout Planner

Week : __________________

Month: __________________

Sunday

Goals

Monday

Goals

Tuesday

Goals

Wednesday

Goals

Thursday

Goals

Friday

Goals

Saturday

Goals

Water Tracker

Mood

Motivation _______________________________________

____

____

____

____

Weekly
Workout Planner

Week :_______________

Month:_______________

Sunday | Monday | Tuesday

Goals | Goals | Goals

Wednesday | Thursday | Friday

Goals | Goals | Goals

Saturday

Water Tracker

Goals

Mood

Motivation

Weekly
Workout Planner

Week : _______________

Month: _______________

Sunday

Monday

Tuesday

Goals

Goals

Goals

Wednesday

Thursday

Friday

Goals

Goals

Goals

Saturday

Water Tracker

Goals

Mood

Motivation _______________________________

____

____

____

____

Weekly
Workout Planner

Week :____________

Month:____________

Sunday   Monday   Tuesday

Goals   Goals   Goals

Wednesday   Thursday   Friday

Goals   Goals   Goals

Saturday   Water Tracker

Goals   Mood

Motivation __________________________________